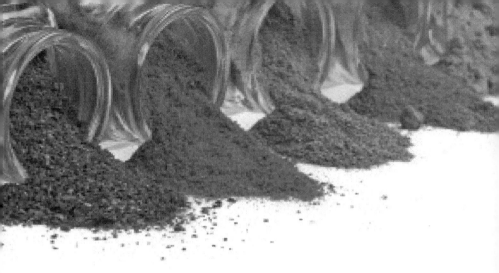

THE

Skinny SLOW COOKER CURRY

RECIPE BOOK

COOKI

D1470838

The Skinny Slow Cooker Curry Recipe Book. Delicious & Simple Low Calorie Curries From Around The World Under 200, 300 & 400 Calories. Perfect For Your Diet Fast Days.

A Bell & Mackenzie Publication
First published in 2014 by Bell & Mackenzie Publishing Limited.

ISBN 978-1-909855-23-6

A CIP catalogue record of this book is available from the British Library

Disclaimer
The information and advice in this book is intended as a guide only. Any individual should independently seek the advice of a health professional before embarking on a diet.

Some recipes may contain nuts or traces of nuts. Those suffering from any allergies associated with nuts should avoid any recipes containing nuts or nut based oils.

Contents

Contents

Contents

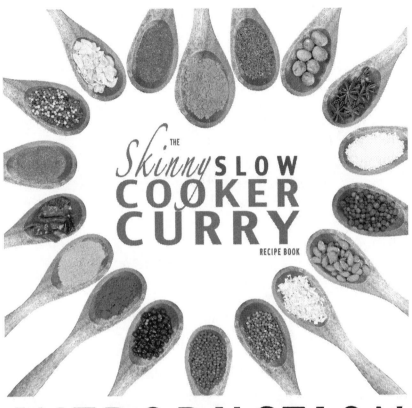

INTRODUCTION

Introduction

Welcome to *The Skinny Slow Cooker Curry Recipe Book* - from the No.1 best selling amazon author of The Skinny Slow Cooker range of recipe books.

Curry has become one of the most loved dishes around the world. Subtle blends of spices that create mouth watering meals reminiscent of the East. Whether you love meat, fish or prefer vegetarian options, there is a curry to suit you. Hot, mild, fragrant, sweet or nutty, the choices are endless. Every country, city and home has their own version of how to make a curry. That's the wonderful thing about cooking with spices, you can experiment to suit your own taste buds and provided you adhere to a few basic principals, you can't really go wrong. While many restaurant style curries are served within minutes of ordering, the slow cooker method allows the full flavour of all the ingredients to penetrate every part of the dish giving maximum flavour to your meal and filling your home with the incredible aroma of a Delhi spice market.

Our recipes are inspired from around the world including more traditional dishes like Korma, Thai Green Curry, Saag Aloo & Rogan Josh, but also a multitude of inspirational easy to prepare curries that will satisfy every palate.

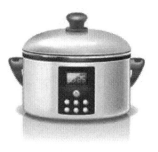

It is easy to be overwhelmed by the idea of cooking curries. With the cuisine relying so heavily on spice blends you can be put off by the vast array on offer before you've even started. Don't be afraid of spices - you'll get to know them quickly and become confident in your cooking in no time. The Skinny Slow Cooker Curry Recipe Book introduces a handful of key spices which you can use time and time again throughout the book and which, once bought, you can keep in the store cupboard and go back to month after month saving you money in the long run.

The slow cooker allows you to prepare delicious curries with the minimum of preparation and fuss. With as little as just 15 minutes preparation you can have a low calorie, nutritious and tasty curry slowly cooking whilst you get on with the things you need to do. If you have a family to cook for, a busy life that means you start early and are out for most of the day, or just don't want to be tied to the kitchen for hours, then the slow cooker is your saviour. Slow cooking enables you to effortlessly prepare meals without worrying that your food will overcook, spill-over or burn. The slow cooking process brings out the best of the ingredients without losing out on goodness. It's easy to use, delivers great results and, with our skinny slow cooker curry recipes, you can be confident you are preparing low calorie & healthy dishes as part of a wholesome diet.

If you have already read one of the other 'Skinny' titles from CookNation, you may be familiar with some of the following information, in which case please feel free to skip straight to our recipes. If however your slow cooker has been stored in a cupboard for months or you have just purchased a slow cooker for the first time, we recommend reading the following pages to familiarise yourself with how to get the best out of your appliance and advice on using our recipes.

During the colder months our bodies naturally crave warm,

filling and comforting food, which can often result in overeating, weight gain and sluggishness.

These delicious curry recipes use simple and inexpensive fresh and store-cupboard ingredients, are packed full of flavour & goodness, and show that you can enjoy maximum taste with minimum calories. All our curry recipes use ingredients that are readily available in most supermarkets so there is no need to source from specialist outlets.

Each recipe has been tried, tested, and enjoyed time and time again. We hope you will find these dishes both delicious and inspirational and perfect to keep count of your calories.

Preparation
All the recipes should take no longer than 10-15 minutes to prepare. Browning the meat will make a difference to the taste of your recipe, but if you really don't have the time, don't worry - it will still taste great.

All meat and vegetables should be cut into even sized pieces unless stated in the recipes. Some ingredients can take longer to cook than others, particularly root vegetables, but that has been allowed for in the cooking time.

As much as possible, meat should be trimmed of visible fat and the skin removed.

Low Cost
Slow cooking is ideal for cheaper meat cuts. The 'tougher' cuts used in this collection of recipes are transformed into

meat which melts-in-your-mouth and helps to keep costs down. We've also made sure not to include too many one-off ingredients, which are used for a single recipe and never used again. All the herbs and spices listed can be used in multiple recipes throughout the book.

Slow Cooker Tips

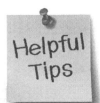

• All cooking times are a guide. Make sure you get to know your own slow cooker so that you can adjust timings accordingly.

• Read the manufacturers operating instructions as appliances can vary. For example, some recommend preheating the slow cooker for 20 minutes before use whilst others advocate switching on only when you are ready to start cooking.

• Slow cookers do not brown meat. While this is not always necessary, if you do prefer to brown your meat you must first do this in a pan with a little low calorie cooking spray.

• A spray of low calorie cooking oil in the cooker before adding ingredients will help with cleaning or you can buy liners.

• Don't be tempted to regularly lift the lid of your appliance while cooking. The seal that is made with the lid on is all part of the slow cooking process. Each time you do lift the lid you may need to increase the cooking time.

• Removing the lid at the end of the cooking time can be useful to thicken up a sauce by adding additional cooking time and continuing to cook without the lid on. On the other hand if the sauce it too thick removing the lid and adding a little more liquid can help.

• Where possible always add hot liquids to your slow cooker, not cold.

• Do not overfill your slow cooker.
• Allow the inner dish of your slow cooker to completely cool before cleaning. Any stubborn marks can usually be removed after a period of soaking in hot soapy water.
• Be confident with your cooking. Feel free to use substitutes to suit your own taste and don't let a missing herb or spice stop you making a meal - you'll almost always be able to find something to replace it.

Our Recipes
The recipes in this book are all low calorie curry dishes serving 4, which makes it easier for you to monitor your overall daily calorie intake as well as those you are cooking for.
The recommended daily calories are approximately 2000 for women and 2500 for men.

Broadly speaking, by consuming the recommended levels of calories each day you should maintain your current weight. Reducing the number of calories (a calorie deficit) will result in losing weight. This happens because the body begins to use fat stores for energy to make up the reduction in calories, which in turn results in weight loss. We have already counted the calories for each dish making it easy for you to fit this into your daily eating plan whether you want to lose weight, maintain your current figure or are just looking for some great-tasting, skinny slow cooker curries.

I'm Already On A Diet. Can I Use These Recipes?
Yes of course. All the curry recipes can be great accompaniments to many of the popular calorie-counting diets. We all know that sometimes dieting can result in

hunger pangs, cravings and boredom from eating the same old foods day in and day out. Our skinny slow cooker curry recipes provide filling meals that should satisfy you for hours afterwards.

I Am Only Cooking For One. Will This Book Work For Me?
Yes. We would recommend following the method for 4 servings then dividing and storing the rest in single size portions for you to use in the future. Most of the recipes will freeze well. Allow all food to cool to room temperature before refrigerating or freezing. When ready to defrost, allow to thaw in a fridge overnight then at room temperature for a few hours depending on the size of the portion. Reheat thoroughly.

Nutrition
All of the recipes in this collection are balanced low calorie meals that should keep you feeling full and help you avoid snacking in-between meals.

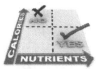

If you are following a diet, it is important to balance your food between proteins, good carbs, dairy, fruit and vegetables.

• **Protein.** Keeps you feeling full and is also essential for building body tissue. Good protein sources come from meat, fish and eggs.
• **Carbohydrates.** Carbs are generally high in calories, which makes them difficult to include in a calorie limiting diet. However carbs are a good source of energy for your body as they are converted more easily into glucose (sugar), providing energy. Try to eat 'good carbs' which are high in

13

fibre and nutrients e.g. whole fruits and veg, nuts, seeds, wholegrain cereals, beans and legumes.
• **Dairy.** Dairy products provide you with vitamins and minerals. Cheeses can be high in calories but other products such as fat free Greek yoghurt, crème fraiche and skimmed milk are all good.
• **Fruit & Vegetables.** Eat your five a day. There is never a better time to fill your 5 a day quota. Not only are fruit and veg healthy, they also fill up your plate and are ideal snacks when you are feeling hungry.

We have adopted the broader nutritional principals in all our recipes.

Portion Sizes
The majority of recipes are for 4 servings. The calorie count is based on one serving. It is important to remember that if you are aiming to lose weight using any of our skinny curry recipes, the size of the portion that you put on your plate will significantly affect your weight loss efforts. Filling your plate with over-sized portions will obviously increase your calorie intake and hamper your dieting efforts.

It is important with all meals that you use a correct sized portion, which is generally the size of your clenched fist. This applies to any side dishes of vegetables and carbs too.

Side Dishes
All the curries in this book fall under 200, 300 & 400 calories. You may choose to serve with a side dish depending on your diet. Traditionally side dishes of bread and rice can be loaded with calories so we have offered a couple of different options.

Each side serves 4. The calories noted are PER SERVING. Here is a guide to those sides:

- 200g/7oz basmati rice **140 calories**
- 200g/7oz fine egg noodles **120 calories**
- 200g/7oz cauliflower rice **50 calories (recipe p.91)**
- 300g/11oz plain green salad **15 calories**

All Recipes Are A Guide Only
All the recipes in this book are a guide only. You may need to alter quantities and cooking times to suit your own appliances.

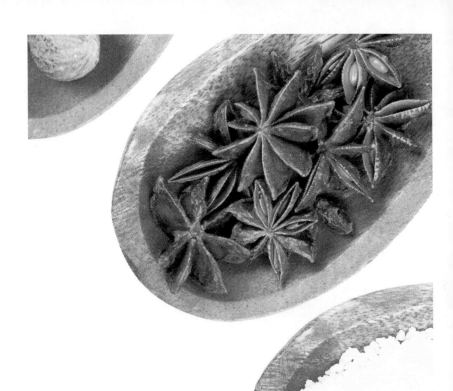

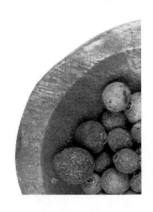

MEAT *The* Skinny SLOW COOKER CURRY RECIPE BOOK

CURRIES

Thai Basil Curry
Serves 4

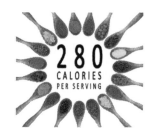

280 CALORIES PER SERVING

Ingredients:

500g/1lb 2oz pork tenderloin, cubed
2 onions, finely chopped
2 tbsp Thai red curry paste
2 tsp tamarind paste
½ tsp ground coriander/ cilantro
1 red pepper, sliced
2 carrots, sliced into batons
1 lemongrass stalk, finely chopped
3 tbsp freshly chopped basil
500ml/2 cups chicken stock/broth
Salt & pepper to taste
Low cal cooking oil spray

Method:

• Season the pork and quickly brown for a couple of minutes in a frying pan with a little low cal oil.
• Remove from the heat and place in the slow cooker along with all the other ingredients.
• Combine well, cover and leave to cook on low for 5-7 hours or until the pork is tender and cooked through.

• For side dish options see page 14

Tamarind paste is made from the tart fruit of the Tamarind tree. It is regularly used in curry as a spicy souring agent.

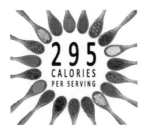

295 CALORIES PER SERVING

Thyme Steak Curry
Serves 4

Method:

• First mix the curry powder and tomato puree together to form a paste.
• Season the steak and quickly brown for a couple of minutes in a frying pan with a little low cal oil.
• Remove from the heat and place in the slow cooker along with all the other ingredients.
Combine well, cover and leave to cook on low for 5-7 hours or until the steak is tender and cooked through.

• For side day options see page 14

You could cook this dish on high for 3-4 hours f you prefer. Reduce the stock by 25% if you do so.

Ingredients:

500g/1lb 2oz lean sirloin steak, thickly sliced
1 tbsp medium curry powder
3 tbsp tomato puree/paste
2 onions, finely chopped
2 garlic cloves, crushed
1 tbsp dried thyme
2 carrots, sliced into batons
150g/5oz sweet potato, diced
2 celery stalks, chopped
500ml/2 cups beef stock/broth
Salt & pepper to taste
Low cal cooking oil spray

Moroccan Lamb & Apricot Curry
Serves 4

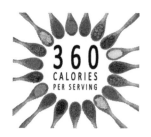

360 CALORIES PER SERVING

Ingredients:

**500g/1lb 2oz lean lamb
fillet, cubed
2 onions, finely chopped
2 garlic cloves, crushed
400g/14oz fresh chopped
tomatoes
100g/3½oz dried apricots,
finely chopped
½ tsp each ground ginger,
turmeric, coriander/
cilantro & paprika
A pinch each of ground
cinnamon, nutmeg & salt
2 carrots, sliced into
batons
120ml/ ½ cup vegetable
stock/broth
Salt & pepper to taste
Low cal cooking oil spray**

Method:

• Season the lamb and quickly brown for a couple of minutes in a frying pan with a little low cal oil.
• Remove from the heat and place in the slow cooker along with all the other ingredients.
• Combine well, cover and leave to cook on low for 5-7 hours or until the lamb is tender and cooked through.

• For side dish options see page 14

Make sure the lamb is trimmed of as much visible fat as possible.

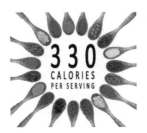

330
CALORIES
PER SERVING

Hot Spiced Creamy Beef Curry
Serves 4

Method:

• Season the beef and quickly brown for a couple of minutes in a frying pan with a little low cal oil.

• Remove from the heat and place in the slow cooker along with all the other ingredients except the Greek yoghurt.

• Combine well, cover and leave to cook on low for 5-8 hours or until the beef is tender and cooked through.

• Add the yoghurt to the slow cooker. Gently stir through and serve.

• For side dish options see page 14

Add a little more beef stock or water during cooking if needed.

Ingredients:

500g/1lb 2oz lean stewing steak, cubed
1 onion, finely chopped
2 garlic cloves, crushed
1 tbsp hot curry powder
2 tbsp tomato puree/paste
2 tsp freshly grated root ginger
½ tsp ground cinnamon (optional)
2 celery stalks, chopped
250ml/1 cup beef stock/ broth
120ml/½ cup fat free Greek yoghurt
Salt & pepper to taste
Low cal cooking oil spray

Pork & Cardamom Curry
Serves 4

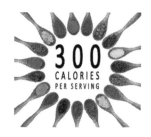

300 CALORIES PER SERVING

Ingredients:

500g/1lb 2oz pork tenderloin, cubed
2 onions, finely chopped
1 red pepper, sliced
2 carrots, sliced into batons
3 garlic cloves, crushed
5 black cardamom pods, crushed
1 tbsp mild curry powder
2 tsp each tamarind paste & cider vinegar
250ml/1 cup chicken stock/broth
120ml/½ cup low fat coconut milk
2 spring onions/scallions, cut into thin ribbons
Salt & pepper to taste
Low cal cooking oil spray

Method:

• Season the pork and quickly brown for a couple of minutes in a frying pan with a little low cal oil.
• Remove from the heat and place in the slow cooker along with all the other ingredients except the coconut milk & spring onions.
• Combine well, cover and leave to cook on low for 4-6 hours or until the pork is tender and cooked through.
• Add the coconut milk to the slow cooker. Gently stir through and serve with the spring onions as a garnish.

• For side dish options see page 14

Cardamon is a highly prized spice. Only saffron and vanilla are more expensive per gram.

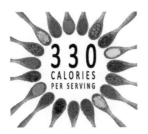

330 CALORIES PER SERVING

Thai Beef Curry
Serves 4

Method:

• Season the steak and quickly brown for a couple of minutes in a frying pan with a little low cal oil.

• Remove from the heat and place in the slow cooker along with all the other ingredients except the coconut cream.

• Combine well, cover and leave to cook on high for 3-5 hours or until the steak is tender and cooked through. Add the coconut cream to the slow cooker. Gently stir through and serve.

• For side dish options see page 14

You could substitute sugar snap peas or mange tout for green beans in this dish if you prefer.

Ingredients:

500g/1lb 2oz lean sirloin steak, thickly sliced
2 tbsp Thai green curry paste
1 red onion, sliced
2 garlic cloves, crushed
1 red pepper, sliced
2 tsp dried basil
1 tbsp each Thai fish sauce, lime juice & soy sauce
250ml/1 cup beef stock/ broth
150g/5oz trimmed green beans
1 tbsp coconut cream
Salt & pepper to taste
Low cal cooking oil spray

Spiced Seed Pork Curry
Serves 4

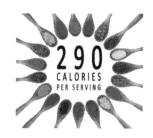

290 CALORIES PER SERVING

Ingredients:

500g/1lb 2oz pork tenderloin, cubed
2 tsp sunflower oil
2 onions, finely chopped
2 garlic cloves, crushed
1 tbsp each cumin & coriander/cilantro seeds
1 red pepper, sliced
1 tbsp medium curry powder
1 tbsp white wine vinegar
1 tsp salt
250ml/1 cup chicken stock/broth
120ml/½ cup low fat coconut milk
2 spring onions/scallions, cut into thin ribbons
Salt & pepper to taste
Low cal cooking oil spray

Method:

• Season the pork and quickly brown for a couple of minutes in a frying pan with a little low cal oil.
• Remove from the heat and place in the slow cooker. Add the sunflower oil, onions, garlic, cumin & coriander seeds to the same frying pan and gently sauté for a few minutes until the seeds begin to pop.
• Add the contents of the pan to the slow cooker along with all the other ingredients except the coconut milk & spring onions.
• Combine well, cover and leave to cook on low for 4-6 hours or until the pork is tender and cooked through. Add the coconut milk to the slow cooker. Gently stir through and serve with the spring onions as a garnish.

• For side dish options see page 14

The cumin and coriander seeds will create a lovely aroma when sautéed to form a fragrant base to the dish.

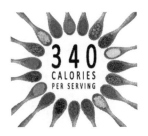

340
CALORIES
PER SERVING

Caribbean Beef Curry
Serves 4

Method:

• Season the steak and quickly brown for a couple of minutes in a frying pan with a little low cal oil.
• Remove from the heat and place in the slow cooker along with all the other ingredients except the coconut cream.
• Combine well, cover and leave to cook on low for 6-8 hours or until the beef is tender and cooked through. Add the coconut cream to the slow cooker. Gently stir through and serve.

Ingredients:

500g/1lb 2oz lean beef stewing steak, cubed
1 tbsp hot curry powder
1 red chilli, finely chopped
1 tbsp tomato puree/paste
400g/14oz tinned chopped tomatoes
2 onions, sliced
3 garlic cloves, crushed
1 tbsp dried thyme
150g/5oz sweet potato, diced
60ml/¼ cup beef stock/broth
1 tbsp coconut cream
Salt & pepper to taste
Low cal cooking oil spray

• For side dish options see page 14

This curry is also nice with a little mixed spice added to give a fragrant finish to the dish.

Beef & Almond Curry
Serves 4

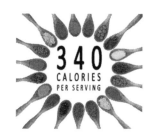

340 CALORIES PER SERVING

Ingredients:

500g/1lb 2oz lean beef stewing steak, cubed
½ tsp each ground turmeric, coriander/cilantro, paprika, ginger, mild curry powder, garam masala & salt
1 red chilli, finely chopped
1 tbsp tomato puree/paste
120ml/ ½ cup tomato passata/sieved tomatoes
1 tbsp ground almonds
2 onions, sliced
3 garlic cloves, crushed
120ml/ ½ cup beef stock/broth
2 tbsp fat free Greek yoghurt
Salt & pepper to taste
Low cal cooking oil spray

Method:

• Season the beef and quickly brown for a couple of minutes in a frying pan with a little low cal oil.
• Remove from the heat and place in the slow cooker along with all the other ingredients except the yoghurt.
• Combine well, cover and leave to cook on low for 6-8 hours or until the beef is tender and cooked through. Add the yoghurt to the slow cooker. Gently stir through and serve.

• For side dish options see page 14

You could use chopped tomatoes rather than passata for this dish if you like.

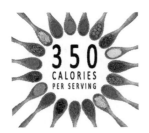

350
CALORIES
PER SERVING

Pea & Beef Curry
Serves 4

Method:

• Season the mince and quickly brown for a couple of minutes in a frying pan with a little low cal oil.
• Remove from the heat and place in the slow cooker along with all the other ingredients.
Combine well, cover and leave to cook on high for 3-5 hours or until the mince is tender and cooked through.

Ingredients:

500g/1lb 2oz lean beef mince
2 onions, sliced
3 garlic cloves, crushed
½ tsp each ground turmeric, cumin, coriander/cilantro, paprika, ginger, medium curry powder, garam masala & salt
1 red chilli, finely chopped
200g/7oz frozen peas
120ml/½ cup tomato passata/sieved tomatoes
60ml/¼ cup beef stock/broth
2 tbsp tomato puree/paste
Salt & pepper to taste
Low cal cooking oil spray

• For side dish options see page 14

This should be a fairly dry dish so leave to cook for longer if necessary.

Korean Beef & Potato Curry
Serves 4

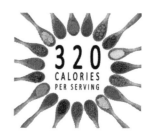

320 CALORIES PER SERVING

Ingredients:

500g/1lb 2oz lean beef
stewing steak
2 onions, sliced
2 garlic cloves, crushed
1 tsp turmeric
½ tsp each ground cumin,
coriander/cilantro, hot
chilli powder & paprika
A pinch of ground ginger,
salt & garam masala
200g/7oz new potatoes,
thickly sliced
200g/7oz spinach leaves
200g/7oz vine ripened
tomatoes, roughly
chopped
120ml/½ cup beef stock/
broth
1 tbsp tomato puree/paste
Salt & pepper to taste
Low cal cooking oil spray

Method:

• Season the beef and quickly brown
for a couple of minutes in a frying pan
with a little low cal oil.
• Remove from the heat and place
in the slow cooker along with all the
other ingredients.
• Combine well, cover and leave to
cook on low for 6-8 hours or until the
beef is tender and cooked through.

• For side dish options see page 14

*Tinned chopped tomatoes are
also fine for this recipe if you
don't have fresh tomatoes to
hand.*

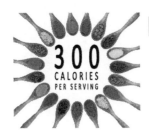

300 CALORIES PER SERVING

Lemongrass & Pork Coconut Curry
Serves 4

Method:

• Season the pork and place in the slow cooker along with all the other ingredients except the coconut milk.

• Combine well, cover and leave to cook on high for 3-5 hours or until the pork is tender and cooked through.

• Remove the curry leaves and add the coconut milk to the slow cooker. Gently stir through and serve.

• For side dish options see page 14

A little freshly chopped coriander makes a nice garnish for this dish.

Ingredients:

500g/1lb 2oz pork tenderloin, diced
2 onions, sliced
2 garlic cloves, crushed
½ tsp each turmeric, ground cumin & coriander/cilantro
1 tbsp medium curry powder
3 lemongrass stalks, finely chopped
5 curry leaves
200g/7oz spinach
2 tbsp tomato puree/paste
180ml/¾ cup vegetable stock/broth
120ml/½ cup low fat coconut milk
Salt & pepper to taste
Low cal cooking oil spray

Beef & Red Pepper Kofta Curry
Serves 4

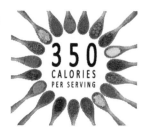

350
CALORIES
PER SERVING

Ingredients:

500g/1lb 2oz lean beef mince
2 garlic cloves, crushed
2 tbsp fresh breadcrumbs
½ tsp each ground turmeric, coriander/cilantro, paprika, ginger, brown sugar, garam masala & salt
1 red chilli, finely chopped
1 onion, sliced
3 red peppers, sliced
250ml/1 cup tomato passata/sieved tomatoes
60ml/¼ cup beef stock/broth
2 tbsp tomato puree/paste
Salt & pepper to taste
Low cal cooking oil spray

Method:

• Place the beef mince, garlic cloves & breadcrumbs in a food processor and pulse a few times until combined.
• Take the mixture out and form into small meatballs with your hands.
• Add all the other ingredients to the slow cooker and place the meatballs on top.
Combine well, cover and leave to cook on high for 4-5 hours or until the meatballs are cooked through.

• For side dish options see page 14

To make breadcrumbs, whizz a slice of bread in a food processor for a few seconds.

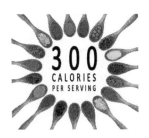

300 CALORIES PER SERVING

Marrakesh Lime & Lamb Curry
Serves 4

Method:

• Season the lamb and quickly brown for a couple of minutes in a frying pan with a little low cal oil.

• Remove from the heat and place in the slow cooker along with all the other ingredients.

Combine well, cover and leave to cook on low for 6-8 hours or until the lamb is tender and cooked through.

Ingredients:

500g/1lb 2oz lean lamb fillet, cubed
2 onions, finely chopped
2 garlic cloves, crushed
400g/14oz fresh chopped tomatoes
Zest & juice of 1 lime
1 tsp each ground turmeric, coriander/cilantro, brown sugar & paprika
½ tsp each ground ginger & hot chilli powder
A pinch of ground cinnamon, nutmeg & salt
120ml/ ½ cup vegetable stock/broth
Salt & pepper to taste
Low cal cooking oil spray

• For side dish options see page 14

Lean neck is a good cut of fillet to use for this curry.

St. Bart's Pork Curry
Serves 4

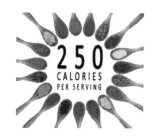

250 CALORIES PER SERVING

Ingredients:

**500g/1lb 2oz pork
tenderloin, cubed
2 onions, finely chopped
1 red pepper, sliced
3 garlic cloves, crushed
150g/5oz butternut squash
flesh, chopped
3 black cardamom pods,
crushed
½ tsp fenugreek seeds
1 tbsp mild curry powder
1 tsp thyme leaves
250ml/1 cup chicken
stock/broth
120ml/½ cup low fat
coconut milk
Salt & pepper to taste
Low cal cooking oil spray**

Method:

• Season the pork and quickly brown
for a couple of minutes in a frying pan
with a little low cal oil.
• Remove from the heat and place in
the slow cooker along with all the other
ingredients except the coconut milk.
• Combine well, cover and leave to
cook on low for 4-6 hours or until the
pork is tender and cooked through.
Add the coconut milk to the slow
cooker. Gently stir through and serve.

• For side dish options see page 14

*Pumpkin or sweet potato
rather than butternut squash
will work just as well in this
curry.*

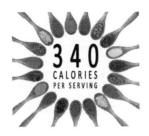

340 CALORIES PER SERVING

Spiced Meatball Curry
Serves 4

Method:

• Place the mince, garlic cloves & breadcrumbs in a food processor and pulse for a few seconds until combined.
• Take the mixture out and form into small meatballs with your hands.
• Add all the other ingredients to the slow cooker and place the meatballs on top.
Combine well, cover and leave to cook on high for 3-5 hours or until the meatballs are cooked through and the cauliflower is tender.

• For side dish options see page 14

You could brown the meatballs first in a frying pan for a few minutes if you have the time.

Ingredients:

500g/1lb 2oz lean pork mince
2 garlic cloves, crushed
2 tbsp fresh breadcrumbs
½ tsp each ground turmeric, coriander/cilantro, paprika, ginger, brown sugar, mild curry powder, garam masala & salt
1 tsp brown sugar
2 red chillies, finely chopped
1 onion, sliced
1 head cauliflower split into florets
250ml/1 cup tomato passata/sieved tomatoes
60ml/¼ cup vegetable stock/broth
2 tbsp tomato puree/paste
Salt & pepper to taste
Low cal cooking oil spray

Hot Bamboo Shoot Beef Curry
Serves 4

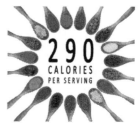

290 CALORIES PER SERVING

Ingredients:

500g/1lb 2oz lean beef stewing steak, cubed
1 tbsp hot curry powder
1 tbsp tomato puree/paste
200g/7oz ready to use bamboo shoots
400g/14oz tinned chopped tomatoes
2 onions, sliced
3 garlic cloves, crushed
1 tbsp dried thyme
60ml/¼ cup beef stock/ broth
1 tbsp coconut cream
Salt & pepper to taste
Low cal cooking oil spray

Method:

• Season the steak and quickly brown for a couple of minutes in a frying pan with a little low cal oil.
• Remove from the heat and place in the slow cooker along with all the other ingredients except the coconut cream.
• Combine well, cover and leave to cook on low for 6-8 hours or until the beef is tender and cooked through.
• Add the coconut cream to the slow cooker. Gently stir through and serve.

• For side dish options see page 14

You could add the bamboo shoots towards the end of cooking if you prefer a little crunch.

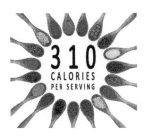

310
CALORIES
PER SERVING

Lamb Jalfrezi
Serves 4

Method:

• Season the lamb and quickly brown for a couple of minutes in a frying pan with a little low cal oil.
• Remove from the heat and place in the slow cooker along with all the other ingredients.
Combine well, cover and leave to cook on low for 5-7 hours or until the lamb is tender and cooked through.

Ingredients:

500g/1lb 2oz lean lamb fillet, cubed
1 onion, finely chopped
2 garlic cloves, crushed
4 green chillies, finely sliced lengthways
½ tsp each cumin, turmeric, paprika, garam masala, ground coriander/cilantro, ginger, cayenne pepper, brown sugar & salt
2 tbsp tomato puree/paste
400g/14oz tinned chopped tomatoes
60ml/¼ cup vegetable stock/broth
Salt & pepper to taste
Low cal cooking oil spray

• For side dish options see page 14

Jalfrezi is a very popular dish, which traditionally contains fresh green chillies.

Beef Madras
Serves 4

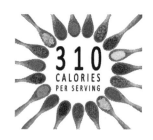

310 CALORIES PER SERVING

Ingredients:

**500g/1lb 2oz lean beef
stewing steak, cubed
2 onions, sliced
2 garlic cloves, crushed
1 tbsp hot curry powder
½ tsp each cumin,
turmeric, ground
coriander/cilantro, brown
sugar & salt
3 tbsp tomato puree/paste
400g/14oz tinned chopped
tomatoes
60ml/¼ cup beef stock/
broth
2 tsp lemon juice
Salt & pepper to taste
Low cal cooking oil spray**

Method:

• Season the beef and quickly brown for a couple of minutes in a frying pan with a little low cal oil.
• Remove from the heat and place in the slow cooker along with all the other ingredients.
Combine well, cover and leave to cook on low for 5-7 hours or until the beef is tender and cooked through.

• For side dish options see page 14

Madras is a hot curry. Feel free to alter the spice to suit your own palate.

POULTRY CURRIES

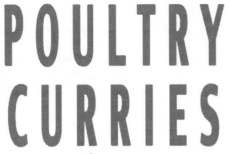

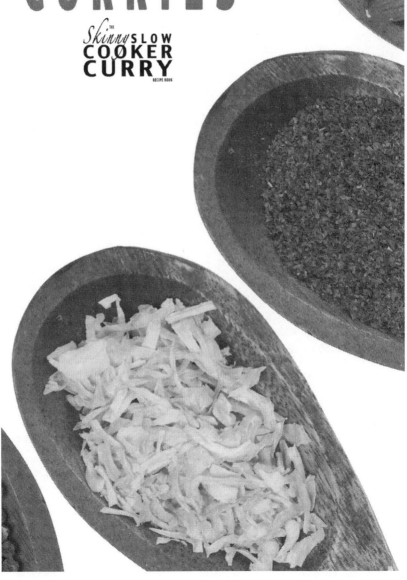

Fiery Chicken Curry
Serves 4

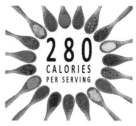

280 CALORIES PER SERVING

Ingredients:

500g/1lb 2oz skinless chicken breast meat, cubed
2 tbsp tomato puree/paste
2 onions, finely chopped
2 garlic cloves, crushed
200g/7oz potatoes, diced
120ml/½ cup chicken stock/broth
250ml/1 cup tomato passata/sieved tomatoes
½ tsp each ground ginger, coriander/cilantro, turmeric, salt & cumin
2 tsp hot chilli powder & brown sugar
Salt & pepper to taste
Low cal cooking oil spray

Method:

• Season the chicken and place in the slow cooker along with all the other ingredients.
Combine well, cover and leave to cook on low for 6-7 hours or until the chicken is tender and cooked through.

• For side dish options see page 14

You could also use cayenne pepper rather than hot chilli powder for this recipe.

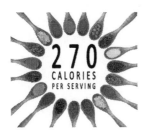

270
CALORIES
PER SERVING

Chicken & Almond Curry
Serves 4

Method:

• Season the chicken and quickly brown for a couple of minutes in a frying pan with a little low cal oil.

• Remove from the heat and place in the slow cooker along with all the other ingredients except the Greek yoghurt.

• Combine well, cover and leave to cook on high for 3-5 hours or until the chicken is tender and cooked through. Add the yoghurt to the slow cooker. Gently stir through and serve.

• For side dish options see page 14

The almonds give this Korma style dish a lovely nutty taste.

Ingredients:

500g/1lb 2oz skinless chicken breast meat, cubed
2 onions, finely chopped
2 garlic cloves, crushed
1 tsp turmeric
½ tsp each ground coriander/cilantro, cumin, paprika, mild chilli powder, ground ginger & salt
1 tbsp ground almonds
1 tbsp tomato puree/paste
180ml/¾ cup chicken stock/broth
120ml/½ cup fat free Greek yoghurt
Salt & pepper to taste
Low cal cooking oil spray

Chicken & Soy Curry
Serves 4

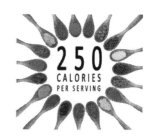

250 CALORIES PER SERVING

Ingredients:

500g/1lb 2oz skinless chicken breast meat, cubed
2 onions, finely chopped
3 garlic cloves, crushed
½ tsp each turmeric, ground ginger, coriander/cilantro, cumin, paprika & chilli powder
2 tbsp tomato puree/paste
1 tsp brown sugar
120ml/½ cup chicken stock/broth
120ml/½ cup soy sauce
Salt & pepper to taste
Low cal cooking oil spray

Method:

• Season the chicken and quickly brown for a couple of minutes in a frying pan with a little low cal oil.
• Remove from the heat and place in the slow cooker along with all the other ingredients.
Combine well, cover and leave to cook on high for 2-4 hours or until the chicken is tender and cooked through.

• For side dish options see page 14

The distinctive flavour of soy sauce is known as 'umami' in Japanese, which means "pleasant savoury taste".

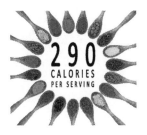

290
CALORIES
PER SERVING

Rogan Josh
Serves 4

Method:

• Season the chicken and quickly brown for a couple of minutes in a frying pan with a little low cal oil.
• Remove from the heat and place in the slow cooker along with all the other ingredients.
Combine well, cover and leave to cook on high for 4-6 hours or until the chicken is tender and cooked through.

• For side dish options see page 14

Ingredients:

500g/1lb 2oz skinless chicken breast meat, cubed
4 onions, sliced
2 garlic cloves, crushed
400g/14oz tinned chopped tomatoes
1 tsp turmeric
½ tsp each garam masala, ground coriander/cilantro, cumin, paprika, hot chilli powder, ground ginger & salt
3 tbsp tomato puree/paste
200g/7oz potatoes, finely chopped
1 tsp brown sugar
60ml/¼ cup chicken stock/ broth
Salt & pepper to taste
Low cal cooking oil spray

This curry should have a thick onion and tomato base. Leave to cook for a little longer if it needs thickening.

41

Chicken & Butternut Squash Curry
Serves 4

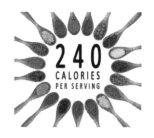

240 CALORIES PER SERVING

Ingredients:

500g/1lb 2oz skinless chicken breast meat, cubed
1 tbsp medium curry powder
2 tbsp tomato puree/paste
2 onions, sliced
2 garlic cloves, crushed
2 tsp dried basil
2 carrots, sliced into batons
150g/5oz butternut squash, diced
2 celery stalks, chopped
250ml/1 cup chicken stock/broth
Salt & pepper to taste
Low cal cooking oil spray

Method:

• Season the chicken and quickly brown for a couple of minutes in a frying pan with a little low cal oil.
• Remove from the heat and place in the slow cooker along with all the other ingredients.
• Combine well, cover and leave to cook on low for 5-7 hours or until the chicken is tender and cooked through.

• For side dish options see page 14

You could use sweet potato rather than butternut squash in this recipe if you prefer.

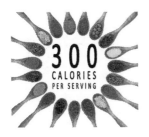

300 CALORIES PER SERVING

Sweet Potato & Chicken Curry
Serves 4

Method:

• Season the chicken and quickly brown for a couple of minutes in a frying pan with a little low cal oil.

• Remove from the heat and place in the slow cooker along with all the other ingredients except the coconut milk.

• Combine well, cover and leave to cook on high for 3-5 hours or until the chicken and sweet potatoes are tender and cooked through.

• Add the coconut milk to the slow cooker. Gently stir through and serve.

• For side dish options see page 14

Add a little more stock during cooking if the dish needs it.

Ingredients:

500g/1lb 2oz skinless chicken breast meat, cubed
1 onion, sliced
2 garlic cloves, crushed
½ tsp each turmeric, ground cumin, coriander/ cilantro, mild chilli powder, ginger, paprika, salt & garam masala
200g/7oz sweet potatoes, cubed
200g/7oz peas
2 tbsp tomato puree/paste
180ml/ ¾ cup chicken stock/broth
120ml/½ cup low fat coconut milk
Salt & pepper to taste
Low cal cooking oil spray

Chicken Keema
Serves 4

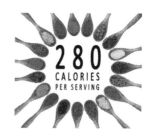

280 CALORIES PER SERVING

Ingredients:

500g/1lb 2oz lean chicken or turkey mince
2 onions, sliced
2 garlic cloves, crushed
½ tsp each turmeric, ground cumin & coriander/cilantro
2 tsp hot curry powder
200g/7oz peas
2 tbsp tomato puree/paste
180ml/¾ cup chicken stock/broth
120ml/½ fat free Greek yoghurt
Salt & pepper to taste
Low cal cooking oil spray

Method:

• Season the mince and quickly brown for a couple of minutes in a frying pan with a little low cal oil.
• Remove from the heat and place in the slow cooker along with all the other ingredients except the yoghurt.
• Combine well, cover and leave to cook on high for 3-5 hours or until the mince is cooked through.
• Add the Greek yoghurt to the slow cooker. Gently stir through and serve.

• For side dish options see page 14

Frozen peas are fine to use for this recipe. Place them in a little boiling water for a minute or two to warm through before adding to the slow cooker.

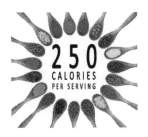

250 CALORIES PER SERVING

Garam Masala Chicken Curry
Serves 4

Method:

• Season the chicken and place in the slow cooker along with all the other ingredients.
• Combine well, cover and leave to cook on low for 4-6 hours or until the chicken is tender and cooked through.

• For side dish options see page 14

Garam masala is a standard shop-bought spice in the west, however its components vary dramatically in Asia where regional variations are commonplace.

Ingredients:

500g/1lb 2oz skinless chicken breast meat, cubed
2 tbsp tomato puree/paste
3 onions, sliced
1 green pepper, sliced
2 garlic cloves, crushed
120ml/½ cup chicken stock/broth
120ml/½ cup tomato passata/sieved tomatoes
2 tsp garam masala
½ tsp each ground coriander/cilantro, turmeric, hot chilli powder, ginger & cumin
2 tsp brown sugar
125g/4oz green beans, chopped
Salt & pepper to taste
Low cal cooking oil spray

Chicken & Tamarind Curry
Serves 4

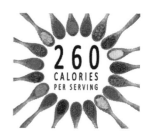

260 CALORIES PER SERVING

Ingredients:

500g/1lb 2oz skinless chicken breast meat, cubed
2 onions, sliced
2 garlic cloves, crushed
½ tsp each turmeric, ground cumin & coriander/cilantro
2 tsp medium curry powder
3 lemongrass stalks, finely chopped
2 tsp tamarind paste
Juice & zest of 1 lime
3 curry leaves
200g/7oz spinach
2 tbsp tomato puree/paste
120ml/½ cup vegetable stock/broth
120ml/½ cup low fat coconut milk
Salt & pepper to taste
Low cal cooking oil spray

Method:

• Season the chicken and place in the slow cooker along with all the other ingredients except the coconut milk.
• Combine well, cover and leave to cook on high for 3-5 hours or until the chicken is tender and cooked through.
• Add the coconut milk to the slow cooker. Gently stir through and serve.

• For side dish options see page 14

Additional lime wedges make a nice garnish for this dish.

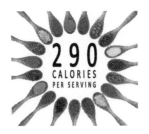

290 CALORIES PER SERVING

Chicken & Mango Curry
Serves 4

Method:

• Season the chicken and place in the slow cooker along with all the other ingredients except the coconut milk.
• Combine well, cover and leave to cook on high for 3-5 hours or until the chicken and mangoes are tender and cooked through.
• Add the coconut milk to the slow cooker. Gently stir through and serve.

• For side dish options see page 14

Ripe mangos are fine to use in this dish. Add them an hour before the end of cooking time so that they don't lose their form.

Ingredients:

500g/1lb 2oz skinless chicken breast meat, cubed
2 onions, sliced
2 garlic cloves, crushed
½ tsp each turmeric, ground cumin & coriander/cilantro
2 tsp medium curry powder
2 tbsp tomato puree/paste
120ml/½ cup chicken stock/broth
120ml/½ cup low fat coconut milk
2 un-ripened mangos, peeled & de-stoned
Salt & pepper to taste
Low cal cooking oil spray

Thai Chicken Pieces
Serves 4

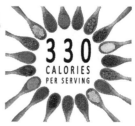

330 CALORIES PER SERVING

Ingredients:

500g/1lb 2oz skinless boneless chicken thighs
2 onions, finely chopped
3 tbsp Thai red curry paste
150g/5oz mushrooms, sliced
4 tbsp freshly chopped coriander/cilantro
1 red pepper, sliced
2 carrots, sliced into batons
250ml/1 cup chicken stock/broth
Salt & pepper to taste
Low cal cooking oil spray

Method:

• Season the chicken and place in the slow cooker along with all the other ingredients.
• Combine well, cover and leave to cook on high for 3-5 hours or until the chicken is tender and cooked through.

• For side dish options see page 14

Reserve a little chopped coriander for garnish.

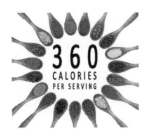

360 CALORIES PER SERVING

Fresh Tomato & Basil Chicken Curry
Serves 4

Method:

• Season the chicken and place in the slow cooker along with all the other ingredients except the coconut cream.
• Combine well, cover and leave to cook on high for 3-5 hours or until the chicken is tender and cooked through.
• Add the coconut cream to the slow cooker. Gently stir through and serve.

• For side dish options see page 14

Dried basil or oregano will also work well in this recipe.

Ingredients:

500g/1lb 2oz skinless boneless chicken thighs, sliced
400g/14oz vine ripened chopped tomatoes
2 onions, sliced
3 garlic cloves, crushed
1 tbsp mild curry powder
2 tbsp tomato puree/paste
1 tsp brown sugar
½ tsp salt
4 tbsp freshly chopped basil
60ml/¼ cup chicken stock/broth
1 tbsp coconut cream
Salt & pepper to taste
Low cal cooking oil spray

'Butter' Chicken
Serves 4

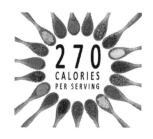

270
CALORIES
PER SERVING

Ingredients:

**500g/1lb 2oz skinless
chicken breast meat,
cubed
2 tbsp low fat olive spread
2 garlic cloves, crushed
½ tsp each ground
turmeric, cumin,
coriander/cilantro,
paprika, ginger, crushed
chilli flakes, garam masala
& salt
1 tsp brown sugar
250ml/1 cup tomato
passata/sieved tomatoes
60ml/¼ cup vegetable
stock/broth
3 tbsp tomato puree/paste
120ml/½ cup fat free
Greek yoghurt
Salt & pepper to taste
Low cal cooking oil spray**

Method:

• Season the chicken and seal for a
couple of minutes in a frying pan with a
little low cal oil.
• Remove from the heat and place in
the slow cooker along with all the other
ingredients except the yoghurt.
• Combine well, cover and leave to
cook on high for 3-5 hours or until the
chicken is tender and cooked through.
• Add the yoghurt to the slow cooker.
Gently stir through and serve.

• For side dish options see page 14

*This is a great 'skinny' version
of the classic calorific dish.*

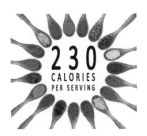

230
CALORIES
PER SERVING

Chicken Bhuna
Serves 4

Method:

• Season the chicken and quickly brown for a couple of minutes in a frying pan with a little low cal oil.
• Remove from the heat and place in the slow cooker along with all the other ingredients except the Greek yoghurt.
• Combine well, cover and leave to cook on high for 3-5 hours or until the chicken is tender and cooked through.
• Add the yoghurt to the slow cooker. Gently stir through and serve.

• For side dish options see page 14

Use any mixture of vegetables you prefer for this classic medium dish.

Ingredients:

500g/1lb 2oz skinless chicken breast meat, cubed
1 onion, finely chopped
250g/9oz mixture of chopped carrots, cauliflower & peas
2 garlic cloves, crushed
½ tsp each cumin, turmeric, paprika, garam masala, medium chilli powder, ground coriander/cilantro, brown sugar & salt
A pinch of cardamom and fenugreek seeds
2 tbsp tomato puree/paste
400g/14oz tinned chopped tomatoes
60ml/ ¼ cup chicken stock/broth
1 tbsp fat free Greek yoghurt
Salt & pepper to taste
Low cal cooking oil spray

Chicken Dopiaza
Serves 4

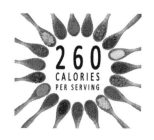

260
CALORIES
PER SERVING

Ingredients:

500g/1lb 2oz skinless chicken breast meat, cubed
4 onions, thickly sliced
2 garlic cloves, crushed
½ tsp each cumin, turmeric, paprika, garam masala, hot chilli powder, ground coriander/cilantro, ginger, brown sugar & salt
2 tbsp tomato puree/paste
180/¾ cup tomato passata/sieved tomatoes
60ml/¼ cup chicken stock/ broth
Salt & pepper to taste
Low cal cooking oil spray

Method:

• Season the chicken and quickly brown for a couple of minutes in a frying pan with a little low cal oil.
• Remove from the heat and place in the slow cooker along with all the other ingredients.
• Combine well, cover and leave to cook on high for 3-5 hours or until the chicken is tender and cooked through.

• For side dish options see page 14

Onions and a thick sauce are the calling cards of this curry.

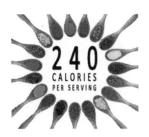

240
CALORIES
PER SERVING

Garlic Chicken
Serves 4

Method:

• Season the chicken and gently sauté for a couple of minutes in a frying pan with a little low cal oil and the sliced garlic.
• Remove from the heat and place in the slow cooker along with all the other ingredients.
• Combine well, cover and leave to cook on high for 3-5 hours or until the chicken is tender and cooked through.

• For side dish options see page 14

Ingredients:

500g/1lb 2oz skinless chicken breast meat, cubed
14 garlic cloves, peeled & finely sliced
1 onion, chopped
½ tsp each cumin, turmeric, paprika, garam masala, hot chilli powder, ground coriander/cilantro, brown sugar & salt
1 tbsp tomato puree/paste
2 vine ripened tomatoes, roughly chopped
180ml/¾ cup tomato passata/sieved tomatoes
60ml/¼ cup chicken stock/broth
Salt & pepper to taste
Low cal cooking oil spray

Be careful not to burn the garlic when you sauté with the chicken. A few drops if water in the pan can help prevent this.

53

Chicken Korma
Serves 4

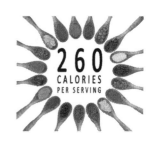

2 6 0
CALORIES
PER SERVING

Ingredients:

**500g/1lb 2oz skinless
chicken breast meat,
cubed
2 garlic cloves, crushed
1 onion, chopped
2 tsp mild curry powder
½ tsp each cumin,
turmeric, paprika & salt
2 tbsp tomato puree/paste
250ml/1 cup tomato
passata/sieved tomatoes
60ml/¼ cup low fat
coconut milk
1 tbsp ground almonds
Salt & pepper to taste
Low cal cooking oil spray**

Method:

• Season the chicken and quickly brown for a couple of minutes in a frying pan with a little low cal oil.
• Remove from the heat and place in the slow cooker along with all the other ingredients except the coconut milk & ground almonds.
• Combine well, cover and leave to cook on high for 3-5 hours or until the chicken is tender and cooked through.
• Add the coconut milk to the slow cooker. Gently stir through and serve with the ground almonds sprinkled over the top.

• For side dish options see page 14

Korma dishes are traditionally 'nutty'. This version contains both coconut milk and ground almonds.

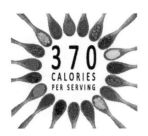

370 CALORIES PER SERVING

Tandoori Chicken
Serves 4

Method:

• Mix together all the ingredients, except the chicken, to form a yoghurt paste.

• Season the chicken and smother with the yoghurt paste.

• Place in the slow cooker, cover and leave to cook on high for 2-4 hours or until the chicken is tender and cooked through.

• For side dish options see page 14

This dish is great served with a simple green salad.

Ingredients:

12 chicken drumsticks
Juice and zest from 1 lemon
2 garlic cloves, crushed
1 tbsp tomato puree/paste
1 tsp mild chilli powder
½ tsp each salt, cumin, turmeric, paprika & black pepper
250ml/1 cup fat free Greek yoghurt
Salt & pepper to taste
Low cal cooking oil spray

Simple Creamy Chicken Curry
Serves 4

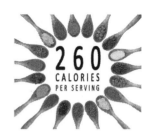

260 CALORIES PER SERVING

Ingredients:

500g/1lb 2oz skinless chicken breast meat, cubed
2 tbsp tomato puree/paste
1 onion, finely chopped
2 garlic cloves, crushed
2 tsp mild curry powder
½ tsp each ground coriander/cilantro, turmeric & cumin
1 tsp brown sugar
120ml/½ cup tomato passata/sieved tomatoes
60ml/ ½ cup chicken stock/broth
60ml/ ½ cup low fat crème fraiche
Salt & pepper to taste
Low cal cooking oil spray

Method:

• Season the chicken and place in the slow cooker along with all the other ingredients except the crème fraiche.
• Combine well, cover and leave to cook on high for 3-5 hours or until the chicken is tender and cooked through.
• Stir through the crème fraiche and serve.

• For side dish options see page 14

This is a really simple, mild curry which should suit everyone's palate.

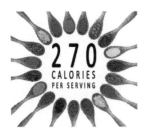

270
CALORIES
PER SERVING

Dhansak
Serves 4

Method:

• Season the chicken and quickly
brown for a couple of minutes in a
frying pan with a little low cal oil.
• Remove from the heat and place
in the slow cooker along with all the
other ingredients except the pineapple
chunks.
• Combine well, cover and leave to
cook on high for 3-5 hours or until the
chicken is tender and cooked through.
• 45 minutes before the end of cooking
add the pineapple chunks to the slow
cooker.
• Season and serve.

• For side dish options see page 14

*You could also use fresh
pineapple for this dish if you
prefer.*

Ingredients:

**500g/1lb 2oz skinless
chicken breast meat,
cubed
2 onions, chopped
2 garlic cloves, crushed
½ tsp each cumin,
turmeric, paprika, garam
masala, ground coriander/
cilantro, ginger, brown
sugar & salt
2 tbsp tomato puree/paste
250ml/1 cup tomato
passata/sieved tomatoes
60ml/ ¼ cup chicken
stock/broth
125g/4oz pineapple
chunks, chopped
Salt & pepper to taste
Low cal cooking oil spray**

Chicken Pasanda
Serves 4

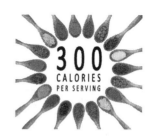

300 CALORIES PER SERVING

Ingredients:

500g/1lb 2oz skinless chicken breast meat, cubed
2 garlic cloves, crushed
1 onion, chopped
1 tbsp mild curry powder
½ tsp salt & brown sugar
3 tbsp tomato puree/paste
250ml/1 cup tomato passata/sieved tomatoes
60ml/¼ cup chicken stock/ broth
60ml/¼ cup fat free Greek yoghurt
2 tbsp chopped cashew nuts
Salt & pepper to taste
Low cal cooking oil spray

Method:

• Season the chicken and quickly brown for a couple of minutes in a frying pan with a little low cal oil.
• Remove from the heat and place in the slow cooker along with all the other ingredients except the yoghurt & cashew nuts. Combine well, cover and leave to cook on high for 3-5 hours or until the chicken is tender and cooked through.
• Meanwhile gently toast the chopped cashew nuts in the frying pan with a little low cal oil for 2-3 minutes until they begin to brown and become fragrant.
• When the chicken is ready add the Greek yoghurt to the slow cooker. Gently stir through and serve with the toasted cashew nuts sprinkled over the top.

• For side dish options see page 14

Toasted almonds also work well for this dish in place of cashew nuts.

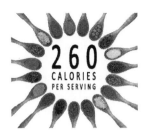

260
CALORIES
PER SERVING

Chicken & Split Pea Curry
Serves 4

Method:

• Place all the ingredients in the slow cooker.
• Combine well, cover and leave to cook on low for 6-8 hours or until the peas & chicken are tender and cooked through.

Ingredients:

500g/1lb 2oz skinless chicken breast meat, cubed
150g/5oz pre soaked split peas
1 tbsp medium curry powder
½ tsp each ground cumin, mustard seeds, salt & brown sugar
2 tbsp tomato puree/paste
370ml/1 ½ cups chicken stock/broth
2 tbsp coconut cream
Salt & pepper to taste
Low cal cooking oil spray

• For side dish options see page 14

Add a little more stock during cooking if the dish needs it.

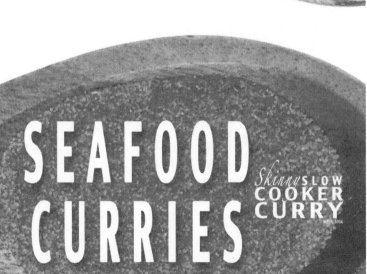

SEAFOOD CURRIES

Skinny SLOW COOKER CURRY RECIPE BOOK

King Prawn Masala
Serves 4

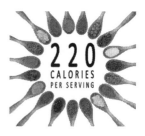

220 CALORIES PER SERVING

Paste Ingredients:
500g/1lb 2oz raw shelled king prawns
2 garlic cloves, crushed
1 tbsp tomato puree/paste
½ tsp each mild chilli powder, salt, cumin, turmeric, paprika & black pepper

Paste Ingredients:
1 onion, chopped
1 tsp cayenne pepper
½ tsp each cumin, turmeric, paprika, garam masala, ground coriander/cilantro & brown sugar & salt
2 tbsp tomato puree/paste
3 vine ripened tomatoes, roughly chopped
180ml/¾ cup tomato passata/sieved tomatoes
60ml/¼ cup chicken stock/broth
120ml/½ cup fat free Greek yoghurt
Lemon wedges to serve
Salt & pepper to taste
Low cal cooking oil spray

Method:

• First mix together the paste ingredients and rub into the king prawns.
• Cover and leave to marinade in a bowl.
• Meanwhile place all the sauce ingredients, except the lemon wedges and Greek yoghurt, in the slow cooker.
• Cover and leave to cook on high for 2 hours.
• Add the prawns and cook for a further 40-70 minutes or until the prawns are cooked through.
• Add the Greek yoghurt and serve with the lemon wedges.

• For side dish options see page 14

Reduce the cayenne pepper in the sauce if your find this dish too spicy for your taste.

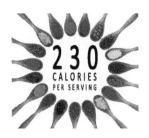

230
CALORIES
PER SERVING

King Prawn & Fresh Pea Curry
Serves 4

Method:

• Place all the ingredients in the slow cooker, except the coconut milk.
• Combine well, cover and leave to cook on high for 3-5 hours or until the prawns are cooked through.
• Add the coconut milk to the slow cooker. Gently stir through and serve.

• For side dish options see page 14

You could hold off adding the fresh peas until 30 mins before the end of cooking if you want them to have a little crunch.

Ingredients:

500g/1lb 2oz raw king prawns
200g/7oz fresh peas
200g/7oz vine ripened tomatoes, roughly chopped
2 garlic cloves, crushed
1 onion, chopped
½ tsp each turmeric, cayenne pepper, cumin, coriander/cilantro, paprika, salt & brown sugar
2 tbsp tomato puree/paste
120ml/½ cup tomato passata/sieved tomatoes
120ml/½ cup low fat coconut milk
Salt & pepper to taste
Low cal cooking oil spray

Paka Hua Alu
Serves 4

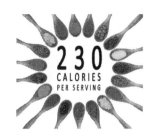

230 CALORIES PER SERVING

Ingredients:

500g/1lb 2oz scallops
150g/5oz spinach
2 garlic cloves, crushed
1 green chilli, finely
chopped
1 onion, sliced
250g/9oz vine ripened
tomatoes, roughly
chopped
½ tsp ground ginger
1 tbsp mild curry powder
60ml/¼ cup fish stock/
broth
12oml/½ cup low fat
crème fraiche
Salt & pepper to taste
Low cal cooking oil spray

Method:

• Place all the ingredients in the slow cooker, except the crème fraiche.
• Combine well, cover and leave to cook on high for 1-3 hours or until the scallops are cooked through.
• Add the crème fraiche, stir & serve.

• For side dish options see page 14

Paka Hua Alu is is the Hindi word for scallops. The fresher the scallops are the better this dish will taste.

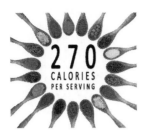

270 CALORIES PER SERVING

Thai Fish Curry
Serves 4

Method:

• Place all the ingredients in the slow cooker, except the coconut milk.
• Combine well, cover and leave to cook on high for 1-3 hours or until the fish is cooked through.
• Add the coconut milk and combine well.

• For side dish options see page 14

Any type of firm white fish will work for this dish. Ensure the bones and skin are removed.

Ingredients:

500g/1lb 2oz firm white fish fillets, cubed
2 garlic cloves, crushed
½ red chilli, finely chopped
2 onions, sliced
Zest and juice of ½ lime
3 tbsp Thai green curry paste
½ tsp ground coriander/ cilantro
120ml/½ cup chicken stock/broth
60ml/¼ cup low fat coconut milk
Salt & pepper to taste
Low cal cooking oil spray

Ginger & Fresh Tomato Prawns
Serves 4

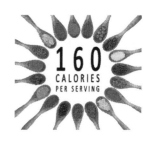

160 CALORIES PER SERVING

Ingredients:

500g/1lb 2oz raw, shelled king prawns
2 tsp freshly grated ginger
½ tsp each turmeric, cumin, coriander/cilantro, paprika, salt & brown sugar
1 red chilli, thinly sliced
200g/7oz vine ripened tomatoes, roughly chopped
2 garlic cloves, crushed
1 onion, sliced
2 tbsp tomato puree/paste
Salt & pepper to taste
Low cal cooking oil spray

Method:

• Mix the prawns, fresh ginger and turmeric together until the prawns are well covered.
• Place all the ingredients in the slow cooker. Combine well, cover and leave to cook on high for 1-3 hours or until the prawns are cooked through.

• For side dish options see page 14

If you don't have fresh ginger use a tsp ground ginger instead.

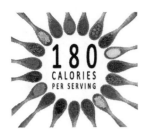

180
CALORIES
PER SERVING

Mackerel Curry
Serves 4

Method:

• Place all the ingredients in the slow cooker.
• Combine well, cover and leave to cook on high for 1-3 hours or until the fish is cooked through.

Ingredients:

500g/1lb 2oz skinless, boneless mackerel fillets
2 garlic cloves, crushed
2 onions, sliced
1 tsp freshly grated ginger
1 tsp cumin seeds
1 tbsp medium curry powder
400g/14oz tinned chopped tomatoes
½ tsp salt & brown sugar
2 tbsp tomato puree/paste
½ red chilli, sliced
Salt & pepper to taste
Low cal cooking oil spray

• For side dish options see page 14

Mackerel a lovely oily fish which is a rich source of essential omega-3 fatty acids.

Coconut Milk & Fish Curry
Serves 4

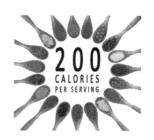

200 CALORIES PER SERVING

Ingredients:

500g/1lb 2oz firm white fish fillets, cubed
½ tsp each ground cumin, turmeric & coriander/ cilantro
2 garlic cloves, crushed
2 red chillies, sliced lengthways
1 onion, sliced
250ml/1 cup low fat coconut milk
2 tbsp freshly chopped coriander/cilantro
Salt & pepper to taste
Low cal cooking oil spray

Method:

• Place all the ingredients in the slow cooker, except the chopped coriander.
• Combine well, cover and leave to cook on high for 1-3 hours or until the fish is cooked through.
• Sprinkle with chopped coriander and serve.

• For side dish options see page 14

Sliced spring onions also make a lovely additional garnish for this dish.

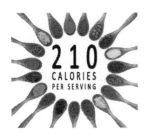

210 CALORIES PER SERVING

Pineapple & Prawn Curry
Serves 4

Method:

• Place all the ingredients in the slow cooker.
• Combine well, cover and leave to cook on high for 1-3 hours or until the prawns are cooked through.

• or side dish options see page 14

The pineapple and tamarind combine well to give a lovely sweet & sour taste.

Ingredients:

500g/1lb 2oz raw, shelled king prawns
½ tsp each turmeric, brown sugar & salt
1 tbsp medium curry powder
2 tsp each fish sauce & tamarind paste
200g/7oz tinned pineapple, chopped
1 lemongrass stalk, finely chopped
2 garlic cloves, crushed
1 onion, chopped
2 tbsp tomato puree/paste
120ml/½ cup low fat coconut milk
Salt & pepper to taste
Low cal cooking oil spray

Fresh Mussel Curry
Serves 4

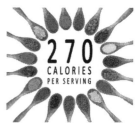

270 CALORIES PER SERVING

Ingredients:

1.kg/3lb 6oz fresh cleaned mussels
2 garlic cloves, crushed
1 onion, chopped
1 tbsp mild curry powder
½ tsp each cumin, turmeric, paprika & salt
2 tbsp tomato puree/paste
250ml/1 cup tomato passata/sieved tomatoes
60ml/¼ cup low fat coconut milk
3 tbsp freshly chopped flat leaf parsley
Salt & pepper to taste
Low cal cooking oil spray

Method:

• Place all the ingredients in the slow cooker, except the chopped parsley.
• Combine well, cover and leave to cook on high for 2-4 hours or until the mussels have opened (discard any which do not open).
• Stir well, sprinkle with parsley and serve in shallow bowls.

• For side dish options see page 14

Buy the freshest mussels possible to get the best result from this dish.

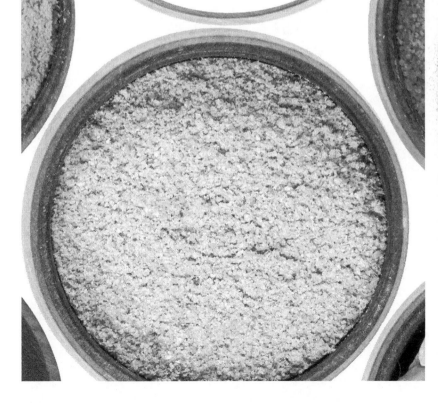

VEGETABLE
CURRIES

The
Skinny SLOW
COOKER
CURRY
RECIPE BOOK

Aloo Gobi
Serves 4

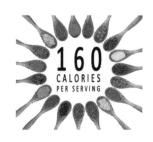

160 CALORIES PER SERVING

Ingredients:

1 large cauliflower head, split into florets
½ green cabbage, shredded
200g/7oz potatoes, cubed
400g/14oz tinned chopped tomatoes
2 garlic cloves, crushed
1 onion, chopped
1 tsp turmeric
½ tsp each cayenne pepper, cumin, coriander/ cilantro, paprika, garam masala, salt & brown sugar
2 tbsp tomato puree/paste
60ml/¼ cup vegetable stock/broth
2 tbsp chopped coriander/ cilantro
Salt & pepper to taste
Low cal cooking oil spray

Method:

• Place all the ingredients in the slow cooker, except the chopped coriander.
• Combine well, cover and leave to cook on high for 3-5 hours or until the vegetables are tender and cooked through.
• Sprinkle with chopped coriander and serve.

• For side dish options see page 14

Spinach and broccoli make good additions to this dish too.

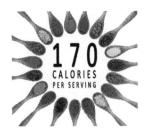

170 CALORIES PER SERVING

Simple Vegetable Curry
Serves 4

Method:

• Place all the ingredients in the slow cooker.
• Combine well, cover and leave to cook on high for 3-5 hours or until the vegetables are tender and cooked through.

Ingredients:

2 carrots cut into batons
1 large cauliflower head, split into florets
200g/7oz spinach leaves
125g/4oz peas
2 onions, chopped
400g/14oz tinned chopped tomatoes
2 garlic cloves, crushed
1 tbsp mild curry powder
½ tsp each salt & brown sugar
2 tbsp tomato puree/paste
60ml/¼ cup vegetable stock/broth
Salt & pepper to taste
Low cal cooking oil spray

• For side dish options see page 14

Add some fresh sliced chillies as a garnish if you want to introduce a little more 'bite' to this dish.

Saag Aloo
Serves 4

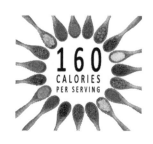

160 CALORIES PER SERVING

Ingredients:

400g/14oz spinach leaves
½ green cabbage,
shredded
200g/7oz potatoes, cubed
2 garlic cloves, crushed
1 onion, chopped
½ tsp each turmeric,
ginger, cumin, coriander/
cilantro, paprika &
mustard seeds
120ml/ ½ cup vegetable
stock/broth
2 tbsp freshly chopped
coriander/cilantro
Lemon wedges to serve
Salt & pepper to taste
Low cal cooking oil spray

Method:

• Place all the ingredients in the slow cooker, except the chopped coriander & lemon wedges.
• Combine well, cover and leave to cook on high for 3-5 hours or until the vegetables are tender and cooked through.
• Sprinkle with chopped coriander, place the lemon wedges on the side and serve.

• For side dish options see page 14

If you have time, you could first quickly sauté the mustard seeds in a little low cal oil for a minute or two until they begin to pop.

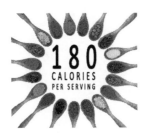

180
CALORIES
PER SERVING

Masaruma & Tomato Curry
Serves 4

Method:

• Place all the ingredients in the slow cooker, except the coconut milk.
• Combine well, cover and leave to cook on high for 3-5 hours or until the vegetables are tender and cooked through.
• Add the coconut milk to the slow cooker. Gently stir through and serve.

• For side dish options see page 14

Ingredients:

500g/1lb 2oz mixed mushrooms, halved
200g/7oz vine ripened tomatoes, roughly chopped
2 garlic cloves, crushed
1 onion, chopped
1 tsp each turmeric, mild chilli powder, cumin, coriander/cilantro, paprika, salt & brown sugar
1 tbsp tomato puree/paste
250ml/1 cup tomato passata/sieved tomatoes
60ml/¼ cup low fat coconut milk
Salt & pepper to taste
Low cal cooking oil spray

If you choose to use large flat mushrooms for this dish they will need to be thickly sliced rather than halved.

Broccoli & Mini Corn Curry
Serves 4

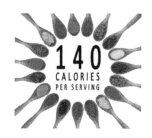

140 CALORIES PER SERVING

Ingredients:

200g/1lb 2oz tenderstem broccoli, halved lengthways
200g/7oz fresh mini corn, left whole
3 carrots, sliced into batons
200g/7oz vine ripened tomatoes, roughly chopped
2 garlic cloves, crushed
1 onion, chopped
½ tsp each turmeric, mild chilli powder, cumin, coriander/cilantro, brown sugar, paprika & salt
2 tbsp tomato puree/paste
120ml/ ½ cup tomato passata/sieved tomatoes
60ml/¼ cup vegetable stock
Salt & pepper to taste
Low cal cooking oil spray

Method:

• Place all the ingredients in the slow cooker.
• Combine well, cover and leave to cook on high for 3-5 hours or until the vegetables are tender and cooked through.

• For side dish options see page 14

Tenderstem broccoli is a lovely seasonal ingredient; use regular fresh broccoli florets if they aren't available.

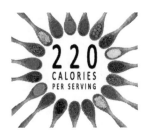

220
CALORIES
PER SERVING

Thai Squash & Coconut Curry
Serves 4

Method:

• Place all the ingredients in the slow cooker, except the coconut milk and lime wedges.

• Combine well, cover and leave to cook on high for 3-5 hours or until the vegetables are tender and cooked through.

• Add the coconut milk to the slow cooker.

• Gently stir through and serve with the lime wedges.

• For side dish options see page 14

Make sure this dish doesn't dry out by adding a little more stock during cooking if needed.

Ingredients:

500g/1lb 2oz butternut squash flesh, cubed
2 onions, finely chopped
3 tbsp Thai red curry paste
½ tsp ground coriander/cilantro
2 carrots, sliced into batons
120ml/½ cup vegetable stock/broth
120ml/½ cup low fat coconut milk
Limes wedges to serve
Salt & pepper to taste
Low cal cooking oil spray

Coriander & Sweet Potato Curry
Serves 4

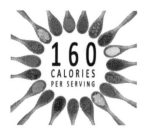

160 CALORIES PER SERVING

Ingredients:

500g/1lb 2oz sweet potatoes, cubed
2 onions, finely chopped
½ tsp each turmeric, mild chilli powder, cumin, coriander/cilantro, paprika & salt
1 red chilli, finely chopped
2 carrots, sliced into batons
120ml/½ cup vegetable stock/broth
120ml/½ cup low fat coconut milk
2 tbsp freshly chopped coriander/cilantro
Lime wedges to serve
Salt & pepper to taste
Low cal cooking oil spray

Method:

• Place all the ingredients in the slow cooker, except the coconut milk, chopped coriander & lime wedges.
• Combine well, cover and leave to cook on high for 3-5 hours or until the vegetables are tender and cooked through.
• Add the coconut milk to the slow cooker. Gently stir through, sprinkle with chopped coriander and serve with the lime wedges.

• For side dish options see page 14

Sweet potatoes are a fantastic versatile vegetable, which form the base of many Caribbean curries.

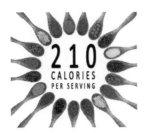

210 CALORIES PER SERVING

Spinach & Paneer
Serves 4

Method:

• Place all the ingredients in the slow cooker, except the crème fraiche & chopped coriander.
• Combine well, cover and leave to cook on high for 3-5 hours or until everything is tender and cooked through.
• Add the crème fraiche to the slow cooker. Gently stir through, sprinkle with chopped coriander and serve.

• For side dish options see page 14

Paneer is the Indian version of cottage cheese, which is now widely available in the UK & US.

Ingredients:

400g/14oz spinach leaves
200g/7oz paneer
200g/7oz vine ripened tomatoes, roughly chopped
2 garlic cloves, crushed
1 onion, chopped
1 tsp each turmeric, cumin, coriander/cilantro, paprika & mustard seeds
½ tsp ground ginger & cayenne pepper
Juice of ½ lemon
60ml/¼ cup vegetable stock/broth
60ml/¼ cup crème fraiche
2 tbsp freshly chopped coriander/cilantro
Salt & pepper to taste
Low cal cooking oil spray

Cumin & Spinach Potatoes
Serves 4

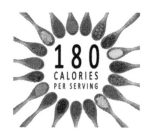

180 CALORIES PER SERVING

Ingredients:

400g/14oz potatoes,
cubed
200g/7oz spinach
1 tsp each ground cumin,
coriander/cilantro &
mustard seeds
½ tsp salt
½ green cabbage,
shredded
120ml/½ cup vegetable
stock/broth
2 tbsp freshly chopped
coriander/cilantro
Lemon wedges to serve
Salt & pepper to taste
Low cal cooking oil spray

Method:

• Place all the ingredients in the slow cooker except the chopped coriander and lime wedges.
• Combine well, cover and leave to cook on high for 3-5 hours or until the potatoes are tender and cooked through.
• Sprinkle with chopped coriander and serve with the lemon wedges.

• For side dish options see page 14

Pointed cabbage rather than savoy cabbage will work best in this recipe.

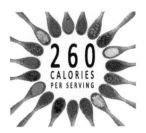

260 CALORIES PER SERVING

Egg Curry
Serves 4

Method:

• Place all the ingredients in the slow cooker, except the coconut milk and eggs.
• Combine well, cover and leave to cook on high for 2 hours.
• Add the boiled eggs and leave to warm through for 30-40 mins.
• Add the coconut milk, combine well and serve.

• For side dish options see page 14

Ingredients:

2 garlic cloves, crushed
2 onions, chopped
2 tsp mild curry powder
½ tsp each cumin, turmeric, paprika & salt
2 tbsp tomato puree/paste
250ml/1 cup tomato passata/sieved tomatoes
8 hardboiled peeled eggs, halved
12oml/½ cup low fat coconut milk
Salt & pepper to taste
Low cal cooking oil spray

Egg curries are a very popular main course in India. Use organic eggs for the best yolks.

Chickpea Curry
Serves 4

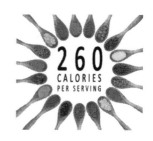

Ingredients:

**600g/1lb 9oz tinned
chickpeas, drained
200g/7oz spinach
2 tsp medium curry
powder
½ tsp ground cumin,
mustard seeds, salt &
brown sugar
2 tbsp tomato puree/paste
250ml/1 cup vegetable
stock/broth
Salt & pepper to taste
Low cal cooking oil spray**

Method:

• Place all the ingredients in the slow cooker.
• Combine well, cover and leave to cook on high for 2-4 hours or until the chickpeas are cooked through.

• For side dish options see page 14

Dried chickpeas are fine to use if they are pre-soaked and prepared.

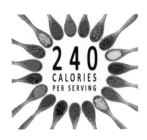

Red Lentil & Courgette Curry
Serves 4

Method:

• Place all the ingredients in the slow cooker.
• Combine well, cover and leave to cook on low for 6-8 hours or until the lentils are tender and cooked through.

• For side dish options see page 14

Add a little more stock during cooking if the lentils require it.

Ingredients:

300g/11oz courgettes/ zucchini thickly sliced
150g/5oz red lentils
2 tsp medium curry powder
½ tsp ground coriander/ cilantro, cumin, mustard seeds, salt & brown sugar
2 tbsp tomato puree/paste
200g/7oz tinned chopped tomatoes
120ml/½ cup vegetable stock/broth
Salt & pepper to taste
Low cal cooking oil spray

Munga Curry
Serves 4

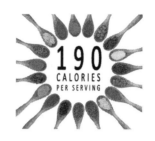

190 CALORIES PER SERVING

Ingredients:

600g/1lb 9oz tinned kidney beans
200g/7oz green beans
1 onion, chopped
2 garlic cloves, crushed
½ tsp each ground coriander/cilantro, mild chilli powder, turmeric, cumin, garam masala & salt
120ml/½ cup vegetable stock/broth
60ml/¼ cup crème fraiche
Salt & pepper to taste
Low cal cooking oil spray

Method:

• Place all the ingredients in the slow cooker.
• Combine well, cover and leave to cook on high for 2-4 hours or until the kidney beans are cooked through.

• For side dish options see page 14

Munga is the Hindi word for kidney beans.

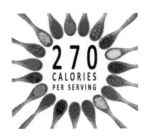

270
CALORIES
PER SERVING

Onion & Egg Masala
Serves 4

Method:

• Place all the ingredients in the slow cooker, except the Greek yoghurt and eggs.
• Combine well, cover and leave to cook on high for 3-4 hours.
• Add the boiled eggs, stir and leave to warm through for 30-40 mins.
• Add the yoghurt, combine well and serve.

• For side dish options see page 14

Slice the onions thickly to give the curry a robust base.

Ingredients:

4 onions, sliced
½ tsp each cumin, turmeric, paprika, garam masala, cayenne pepper, ground coriander/cilantro, brown sugar, ginger & salt
2 tbsp tomato puree/paste
3 vine ripened tomatoes, roughly chopped
250ml/1 cup tomato passata/sieved tomatoes
60ml/¼ cup chicken stock/ broth
4 hardboiled eggs, peeled & halved
120ml/½ cup fat free Greek yoghurt
Salt & pepper to taste
Low cal cooking oil spray

Aloo Cauliflower Curry
Serves 4

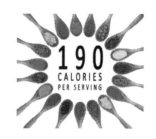

190 CALORIES PER SERVING

Ingredients:

1 large cauliflower heads, split into florets
1 green pepper, sliced
125g/4oz peas
1 onion, chopped
200g/7oz tinned chopped tomatoes
2 garlic cloves, crushed
½ tsp each turmeric, cayenne pepper, cumin, coriander/cilantro & paprika
1 tbsp tomato puree/paste
60ml/¼ cup vegetable stock/broth
4 tbsp freshly chopped flat leaf parsley
Salt & pepper to taste
Low cal cooking oil spray

Method:

• Place all the ingredients in the slow cooker.
• Combine well, cover and leave to cook on high for 3-5 hours or until the vegetables are tender and cooked through.

• For side dish options see page 14

Hold back a little of the parsley as a garnish.

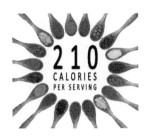

Plantain & Sweet Onion Curry
Serves 4

Method:

• Place all the ingredients in the slow cooker, except the coconut milk.
• Combine well, cover and leave to cook on high for 3-5 hours or until the plantain is tender and cooked through.
• Add the coconut milk, stir and serve.

Ingredients:

2 plantain, peeled & thickly sliced
250g/9oz shallots, halved
2 tsp mild curry powder
½ tsp each cumin, turmeric, paprika, salt, ground cinnamon & brown sugar
2 tbsp tomato puree/paste
125g/4oz vine ripened tomatoes, roughly chopped
120ml/ ½ cup vegetable stock/broth
12oml/½ cup low fat coconut milk
Salt & pepper to taste
Low cal cooking oil spray

• For side dish options see page 14

Plantain is a West Indian vegetable, which is now widely available in the UK & US.

Garlic Curry
Serves 4

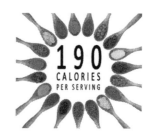

190 CALORIES PER SERVING

Ingredients:

1 whole bulb garlic,
separated & peeled
2 green chillies, finely
chopped
2 tsp tamarind paste
150g/5oz tenderstem
broccoli
2 onions, roughly chopped
5 curry leaves
½ tsp each fennel seeds,
turmeric, cayenne pepper,
salt & brown sugar
2 tbsp tomato puree/paste
125g/4oz vine ripened
tomatoes, roughly
chopped
120ml/½ cup vegetable
stock/broth
12oml/½ cup low fat
crème fraiche
Salt & pepper to taste
Low cal cooking oil spray

Method:

• Place all the ingredients in the slow cooker, except the crème fraiche.
• Combine well, cover and leave to cook on high for 4-6 hours.
• Add the crème fraiche and combine well.
• Remove the curry leaves and serve.

• For side dish options see page 14

This curry is great served with a simple green salad.

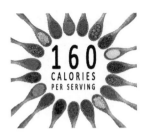

160 CALORIES PER SERVING

Gobhi Coconut Curry
Serves 4

Method:

• Place all the ingredients in the slow cooker, except the desiccated coconut.
• Combine well, cover and leave to cook on high for 3-5 hours or until the vegetables are tender and cooked through.
• Meanwhile heat a dry frying pan and toast the coconut gently until golden brown.
• When the cabbage is ready, sprinkle with the toasted coconut and serve.

Ingredients:

1 large pointed green cabbage, shredded
1 green pepper, thinly sliced
2 green chillies, finely chopped
2 onions, thinly sliced
½ tsp each mustard seeds, turmeric & cumin
250ml/1 cup vegetable stock/broth
75g/3oz desiccated coconut
Salt & pepper to taste
Low cal cooking oil spray

• For side dish options see page 14

Shake the pan continuously to move the coconut around when you are toasting it.

Green Beans & Fenugreek Curry
Serves 4

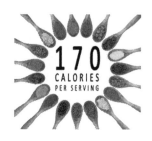

170 CALORIES PER SERVING

Ingredients:

400g/14oz green beans, trimmed & split lengthways
1 red pepper, chopped
2 red chillies, finely chopped
2 onions, thinly sliced
½ tsp each fenugreek seeds, salt & turmeric
120ml/ ½ cup vegetable stock/broth
60ml/¼ cup coconut cream
Lime wedges to serve
Salt & pepper to taste
Low cal cooking oil spray

Method:

• Place all the ingredients in the slow cooker, except the coconut cream and lime wedges.
• Combine well, cover and leave to cook on high for 2-4 hours or until the beans are tender and cooked through.
• Add the coconut cream, stir & serve with the lime wedges.

• For side dish options see page 14

Widely used in Indian cooking, fenugreek seeds are believed to help fend off the common cold!

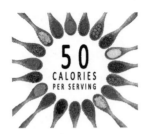

50
CALORIES
PER SERVING

Cauliflower 'Rice'
Serves 4

Method:

• Split the cauliflower head into florets and place in a food processor.
• Whizz until the cauliflower is the size of rice grains.
• Place the 'rice' in a microwavable dish and cook covered for 4-5 minutes or until the 'rice' is piping hot.

Ingredients:

1 large cauliflower head (approx. 800g)

This is a great alternative to rice if you are trying to keep the calories down. It freezes well too, so make a batch and freeze into portions.

CONVERSION CHART: DRY INGREDIENTS

Metric	Imperial
7g	¼ oz
15g	½ oz
20g	¾ oz
25g	1 oz
40g	1½oz
50g	2oz
60g	2½oz
75g	3oz
100g	3½oz
125g	4oz
140g	4½oz
150g	5oz
165g	5½oz
175g	6oz
200g	7oz
225g	8oz
250g	9oz
275g	10oz
300g	11oz
350g	12oz
375g	13oz
400g	14oz

Metric	Imperial
425g	15oz
450g	1lb
500g	1lb 2oz
550g	1¼lb
600g	1lb 5oz
650g	1lb 7oz
675g	1½lb
700g	1lb 9oz
750g	1lb 11oz
800g	1¾lb
900g	2lb
1kg	2¼lb
1.1kg	2½lb
1.25kg	2¾lb
1.35kg	3lb
1.5kg	3lb 6oz
1.8kg	4lb
2kg	4½lb
2.25kg	5lb
2.5kg	5½lb
2.75kg	6lb

CONVERSION CHART: LIQUID MEASURES

Metric	Imperial	US
25ml	1fl oz	
60ml	2fl oz	¼ cup
75ml	2½ fl oz	
100ml	3½fl oz	
120ml	4fl oz	½ cup
150ml	5fl oz	
175ml	6fl oz	
200ml	7fl oz	
250ml	8½ fl oz	1 cup
300ml	10½ fl oz	
360ml	12½ fl oz	
400ml	14fl oz	
450ml	15½ fl oz	
600ml	1 pint	
750ml	1¼ pint	3 cups
1 litre	1½ pints	4 cups

Other
COOKNATION
TITLES

If you enjoyed 'The Skinny Slow Cooker Curry Recipe Book' we'd really appreciate your feedback. Reviews help others decide if this is the right book for them so a moment of your time would be appreciated.

Thank you.

You may also be interested in other '**Skinny**' titles in the CookNation series. You can find all the following great titles by searching under '**CookNation**'.

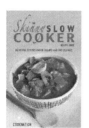

The Skinny Slow Cooker Recipe Book

Delicious Recipes Under 300, 400 And 500 Calories.

Paperback / eBook

More Skinny Slow Cooker Recipes

75 More Delicious Recipes Under 300, 400 & 500 Calories.

Paperback / eBook

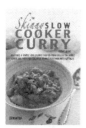

The Skinny Slow Cooker Curry Recipe Book

Low Calorie Curries From Around The World

Paperback / eBook

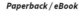

The Skinny Slow Cooker Soup Recipe Book

Simple, Healthy & Delicious Low Calorie Soup Recipes For Your Slow Cooker. All Under 100, 200 & 300 Calories.

Paperback / eBook

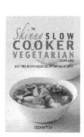

The Skinny Slow Cooker Vegetarian Recipe Book

40 Delicious Recipes Under 200, 300 And 400 Calories.

Paperback / eBook

The Skinny 5:2 Slow Cooker Recipe Book

Skinny Slow Cooker Recipe And Menu Ideas Under 100, 200, 300 & 400 Calories For Your 5:2 Diet.

Paperback / eBook

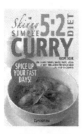

The Skinny 5:2 Curry Recipe Book

Spice Up Your Fast Days With Simple Low Calorie Curries, Snacks, Soups, Salads & Sides Under 200, 300 & 400 Calories

Paperback / eBook

The Skinny Halogen Oven Family Favourites Recipe Book

Healthy, Low Calorie Family Meal-Time Halogen Oven Recipes Under 300, 400 and 500 Calories

Paperback / eBook

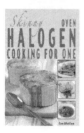

Skinny Halogen Oven Cooking For One

Single Serving, Healthy, Low Calorie Halogen Oven Recipes Under 200, 300 and 400 Calories

Paperback / eBook

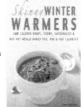

Skinny Winter Warmers Recipe Book

Soups, Stews, Casseroles & One Pot Meals Under 300, 400 & 500 Calories.

Paperback / eBook

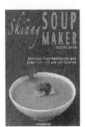

The Skinny Soup Maker Recipe Book

Delicious Low Calorie, Healthy and Simple Soup Recipes Under 100, 200 and 300 Calories. Perfect For Any Diet and Weight Loss Plan.

Paperback / eBook

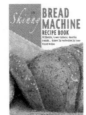

The Skinny Bread Machine Recipe Book

70 Simple, Lower Calorie, Healthy Breads...Baked To Perfection In Your Bread Maker.

Paperback / eBook

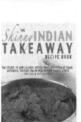

The Skinny Indian Takeaway Recipe Book

Authentic British Indian Restaurant Dishes Under 300, 400 And 500 Calories. The Secret To Low Calorie Indian Takeaway Food At Home

Paperback / eBook

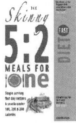

The Skinny Juice Diet Recipe Book

5lbs, 5 Days. The Ultimate Kick-Start Diet and Detox Plan to Lose Weight & Feel Great!

Paperback / eBook

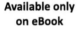

The Skinny 5:2 Diet Recipe Book Collection

All The 5:2 Fast Diet Recipes You'll Ever Need. All Under 100, 200, 300, 400 And 500 Calories

Available only on eBook

eBook

The Skinny 5:2 Fast Diet Meals For One

Single Serving Fast Day Recipes & Snacks Under 100, 200 & 300 Calories

Paperback / eBook

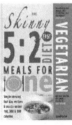

The Skinny 5:2 Fast Diet Vegetarian Meals For One

Single Serving Fast Day Recipes & Snacks Under 100, 200 & 300 Calories

Paperback / eBook

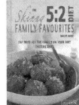

The Skinny 5:2 Fast Diet Family Favourites Recipe Book

Eat With All The Family On Your Diet Fasting Days

Paperback / eBook

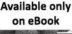

The Skinny 5:2 Fast Diet Family Favorites Recipe Book *U.S.A. EDITION*

Dine With All The Family On Your Diet Fasting Days

Available only on eBook

Paperback / eBook

The Skinny 5:2 Diet Chicken Dishes Recipe Book

Delicious Low Calorie Chicken Dishes Under 300, 400 & 500 Calories

Paperback / eBook

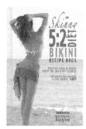

The Skinny 5:2 Bikini Diet Recipe Book

Recipes & Meal Planners Under 100, 200 & 300 Calories. Get Ready For Summer & Lose Weight...FAST!

Paperback / eBook

Available only on eBook

The Paleo Diet For Beginners Slow Cooker Recipe Book

Gluten Free, Everyday Essential Slow Cooker Paleo Recipes For Beginners

eBook

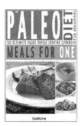

The Paleo Diet For Beginners Meals For One

The Ultimate Paleo Single Serving Cookbook

Paperback / eBook

Available only on eBook

The Paleo Diet For Beginners Holidays

Thanksgiving, Christmas & New Year Paleo Friendly Recipes

eBook

Available only on eBook

The Healthy Kids Smoothie Book

40 Delicious Goodness In A Glass Recipes for Happy Kids.

eBook

The Skinny Slow Cooker Summer Recipe Book

Fresh & Seasonal Summer Recipes For Your Slow Cooker. All Under 300, 400 And 500 Calories.

Paperback / eBook

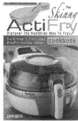

The Skinny ActiFry Cookbook

Guilt-free and Delicious ActiFry Recipe Ideas: Discover The Healthier Way to Fry!

Paperback / eBook

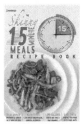

The Skinny 15 Minute Meals Recipe Book

Delicious, Nutritious & Super-Fast Meals in 15 Minutes Or Less. All Under 300, 400 & 500 Calories.

Paperback / eBook

The Skinny Mediterranean Recipe Book

Simple, Healthy & Delicious Low Calorie Mediterranean Diet Dishes. All Under 200, 300 & 400 Calories.

Paperback / eBook

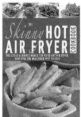

The Skinny Hot Air Fryer Cookbook

Delicious & Simple Meals For Your Hot Air Fryer: Discover The Healthier Way to Fry.

Paperback / eBook

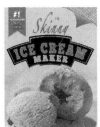

The Skinny Ice Cream Maker

Delicious Lower Fat, Lower Calorie Ice Cream, Frozen Yogurt & Sorbet Recipes For Your Ice Cream Maker

Paperback / eBook

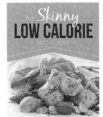

The Skinny Low Calorie Recipe Book

Great Tasting, Simple & Healthy Meals Under 300, 400 & 500 Calories. Perfect For Any Calorie Controlled Diet.

Paperback / eBook

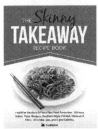

The Skinny Takeaway Recipe Book

Healthier Versions Of Your Fast Food Favourites: Chinese, Indian, Pizza, Burgers, Southern Style Chicken, Mexican & More. All Under 300, 400 & 500 Calories

Paperback / eBook

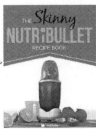

The Skinny Nutribullet Recipe Book

80+ Delicious & Nutritious Healthy Smoothie Recipes. Burn Fat, Lose Weight and Feel Great!

Paperback / eBook

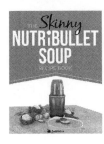

The Skinny Nutribullet Soup Recipe Book

Delicious, Quick & Easy, Single Serving Soups & Pasta Sauces For Your Nutribullet. All Under 100, 200, 300 & 400 Calories.

Paperback / eBook

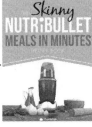

The Skinny Nutribullet Meals In Minutes Recipe Book

Quick & Easy, Single Serving Suppers, Snacks, Sauces, Salad Dressings & More Using Your Nutribullet. All Under 300, 400 & 500 Calories.

Paperback / eBook

19594279R00058

Printed in Poland
by Amazon Fulfillment
Poland Sp. z o.o., Wrocław